STRENGTH AND N

The Ultimate 26-Week Guide to Building Life-Cha

Power.

Jason Farley

Copyright

Legal Disclaimer

The information presented in this work is by no way intended as medical advice or as a substitute for medical counseling. The information should be used in conjunction with the guidance and care of your physician. Consult your physician before beginning this program. This program is designed for healthy individuals 18 years and older only. Perform these exercises at your own risk. By continuing with the program, you expressly assume such risks and waive future physical injury while lifting or moving weights at your gym, home or elsewhere. You also relinquish and release any claim that you may have against Jason Farley or his affiliates as a result of any illness incurred in connection with, or as a result of, the use or misuse of the program

TABLE OF CONTENTS

WELCOME.

First off, I'd like to thank you for purchasing my book, Strength and Mass. Within the following pages lies the blueprint to achieving a phenomenally aesthetic and strong physique. You will command respect and attention wherever you go, the guys will want to be you and the girls will want to be with you. As your body grows, so will your confidence and your outlook on life. You will become a true alpha.

Strength and Mass is a 26-week periodized training program. The overall goal of the program as you may have guessed is to help you build the maximum amount of muscle and strength over the coming 6 months as is humanely possible. The strategies and techniques you will learn during this journey can be used well after the program has finished to allow you to continue to build and mould your body into one of your dreams. Whatever your goals are, this program can help you obtain real results without using performance-enhancing drugs, spending a ton on supplements, or wasting extra time in the gym. All the information you need to build the body of your dreams lies within these pages

I designed this book to empower you; you won't find cookie filler content, a basic workout program that a monkey could have designed, and you wont find links to buy my "recommended" supplements. What you will find is good, old fashioned, no-nonsense advice.

The journey to a strong and aesthetic physique is not going to be an easy one; you will have to make sacrifices along the way (some easier than others) but I promise you that if you commit yourself fully to this program, you will see results. You will finally be able to look in the mirror and beam with pride at what you have created. So I urge you now - grab life by the balls, take action and reap the rewards!

Have a great workout!

Jason Farley

CHAPTER 1: HOW IS MUSCLE BUILT?

So many people throw themselves into training, just going through the motions, just doing what they're told. Sure I could just tell you to do 3 sets of 10 and assure you that it's going to work but what would you be able to take away? What would you actually learn? You want bigger muscles? Fine. But in order to fully understand why this program as been designed this way, you must first understand how muscle is built.

What makes a muscle grow?

There are three main mechanisms involved in producing muscle growth. Many basic workout programs limit you to using one or perhaps two mechanisms, which isn't optimal if you're looking to maximize your results in the shortest time frame. All three of the mechanisms below must be implemented into your regime:

1) Mechanical Tension

Mechanical tension refers to stress placed on a muscle through large amounts of tension (A muscle generates tension by contracting). This is where progressive overload comes in; it is the cornerstone behind every successful workout plan. Progressive overload is the process whereby you gradually lift heavier and heavier weights overtime, thereby increasing the amount of tension running through the muscles. The muscle adapts to the increased stress by growing more muscle. In order to fully maximize mechanical tension, you have to lift heavier weights in a lower rep range.

2) Muscle Damage

Muscle damage is when your training creates small micro-tears in your muscles thus signalling your body to repair it. With proper nutrition and rest, the body will repair these micro-tears causing the muscle fibres to grow bigger in order to better deal with the stresses you're placing on it.

3) Metabolic Stress

Metabolic stress is caused by cell swelling around your muscle, which your muscles cells sense as a threat so they grow. Everyone's favourite feeling at the gym causes metabolic stress, or *the Pump*. The best way to train for metabolic stress is by training in higher rep-ranges and shorter rest periods to maximize the amount of cell swelling in your muscle. The problem with most basic workout programs is that they generally emphasise metabolic stress. Common advice with most of these programs is "train in the 8 -12 rep range and go to failure". The problem however lies in the fact that most of these programs are not based around progressive overload, which can be hard to induce when you're always training in the higher rep-ranges.

The two main types of muscle growth

There seems to be two main hypertrophic responses to training. Training in different ways emphasises different types of muscle growth.

1) Sarcoplasmic Hypertrophy

Sarcoplasmic hypertrophy is a hypertrophic (growth) response whereby there is an increase of muscle cell fluid or sarcoplasm within a muscle cell. Since the fluid contains non-contractile elements such as water, glycogen etc. you won't gain much real strength from this alone. However the upside to this is that as it's fluid, it's a much faster way to increase the size of a muscle.

2) Myofibrillar hypertrophy

Myofibrillar hypertrophy is a hypertrophic (growth) response whereby there is an increase in the size of the muscle fibers. As it's an actual increase in the size of the muscle fibers, myofibrillar hypertrophy mainly causes an increase in strength. However in terms of building size, it's a much slower process.

So the takeaway lesson here is essentially that lifting heavier in lower rep-ranges emphasizes myofibrillar hypertrophy and lifting lighter weights in a higher rep-range emphasizes sarcoplasmic hypertrophy. In order to fully maximize strength and muscle growth you need to induce both types of hypertrophy and progressively overload your muscles in all rep-ranges.

Chapter 2: How to ensure progressive overload

As I briefly mentioned earlier, progressive overload is the method of gradually increasing the demands placed on your muscles. This is the foundation behind the Size and Strength training program. To get bigger and stronger you must induce progressive overload every workout. This is why so many people simply don't progress, as without it, there is no reason for your body to adapt and therefore no reason for your body to build muscle.

Three proven ways to induce progressive overload

There are lots more ways to induce progressive overload but these three seem to be the most practical.

1) Increase of resistance

A good indicator that you're inducing progressive overload is by an increase in the weights that you use within your target rep ranges.

2) Increase of repetitions (providing weight is the same)

If you do more reps with the same weight, you have become stronger. If you can do more reps than the target rep-range, than it's time to increase the weights!

3) Increase of Sets (providing weight is the same)

By increasing the amount of sets done on a particular muscle group, you are increasing the total training volume and also the amount of work done by the muscle. The muscle will therefore have to adapt to the new stresses.

CHAPTER 3: THE TOP COMMANDMENTS OF BUILDING MUSCLE

"The Iron never lies to you. You can walk outside and listen to all kinds of talk, get told that you're a god or a total bastard. The Iron will always kick you in the real deal. The Iron is the great reference point, the all-knowing perspective giver, always there like a beacon in the pitch black. I have found the iron to be my greatest friend. It never freaks out on me, never runs. Friends may come and go. But two hundred pounds is always two hundred pounds" -Henry Rollins

So you have read the science, now let's put this into practice.

1) You must lift heavy (as dictated by the rep-ranges).

As a natural lifter, this is the most powerful way of building solid muscle. If anyone tells you that you can build muscle by lifting light weights, just tell them they're a pussy. Think about it, if weight didn't matter, you could grow just by curling a can of baked beans. I can guarantee that if you are still benching the same as you did 5 months ago, then your chest still looks the same. You simply cannot grow any significant amount of muscle without forcing your muscles to adapt to a greater stimulus. Think about it, have you ever seen someone who deadlifts 500 pounds who still has small arms? Probably not. The only way to build real hard dense muscle is with heavy weights.

2) You must progressively overload the muscle.

Your muscles will only grow if they're forced too. By progressively overloading the muscle, you are consistently forcing your muscles to adapt to new stimulus and therefore, build more muscle to handle that stimulus. On the other hand, if the stresses placed on your muscles are not at least maintained or are decreased, your muscle will adapt to that and in turn you will lose muscle. If you take anything away from this book let it be this. - you must always beat your last workout. Always strive for a new personal best (PB) each and every workout.

3) You must let your muscles recover (take days off).

Your muscles do not grow in the gym; they grow with adequate rest. So many hard-core bodybuilding programs have you hit your muscles too frequently; this in turn leads to little to no muscle gains. Without letting your muscle fully recover you will be unable to apply progressive overload and this can lead to you plateauing or losing you hard-earned muscle. You must also make sure you get enough sleep, as this is when the growth occurs. For most people this means getting about 8-10 hours of sleep a day.

4) You must supply them with the right building blocks to grow

What are those building blocks? Well food of course. But not any type of food, otherwise you could build muscle just eating chocolate bars and ice cream. You can have the best training program in the world, but if you aren't supplying your body with enough calories, you simply won't grow. In order to build muscle, you have to be in a calorie surplus. However, you do not want to make the mistake that most misguided individuals make and fill that with pizzas and chips, because doing so on a long-term basis is extremely unhealthy. You want to fill it with clean calories and nutrient dense foods like eggs, fish, fruit, and vegetables.

5) Base your workouts around compound movements

Compound movements are exercises that recruit more than one muscle group. They recruit more muscle fibres and allow you to use heavier loads. In addition they will lead to the biggest release of anabolic hormones in your body leading to, you guessed it – more muscle growth. Now I love bicep curls as much as the next man and of course they have their place in a well designed program but since compound movements give you the most bang for your buck, they should be your priority. Examples of compound movements would be the bench press, squat or deadlift.

6) Train in a variety of rep-ranges

This is where so many people and workout programs go wrong; they stick to the same rep-ranges for months on end. In order to fully maximize your training results you must vary the rep-ranges to insure you create myofibrillar and sarcoplasmic growth.

As you can see, there's no secret method to building eye-popping quality muscle, that's just what the magazines and supplement companies want you to believe. Building quality muscle isn't hard; it just takes time, more than most people are willing to wait for. Building the body of your dreams is a simple as this: train heavy, eat smart, sleep, and repeat.

Yeah it's really that simple.

CHAPTER 4: THE TOP REASONS HOLDING OTHERS BACK FROM THE BODY OF THEIR DREAMS

You see them in the gym all the time, the guys that have been there for years, slaving away at the weights, always trying new workout routines, novel exercises and the latest newly hyped supplements but one thing always remains the same: them. They look no different from when they started. They are your average Joe "gym goer" and they all seem to make the same mistakes. They're also the same people to accuse everyone with greater muscularity then them that they're on 'roids. So before you get started with the program, if you don't want to be that guy, 5 years from now who still looks the same, then heed the warnings below.

1) Not setting goals

The ultimate reason that most people fail or quit is simply because they didn't have a definable target to aim for when they got started. So many people start off training with such vague goals like "I want bigger arms" or "I want to have a six pack" but so few actually define them. If you only take one thing away from this book that will help more than any other training program or new supplement is this: set definable goals. Simply saying you want bigger arms is not enough - actually set a measurement target e.g. 16 inches and commit to it. The ultimate reason that most people fail or quit is simply because they didn't have a definable target to aim for. You must also set a deadline in which you want to achieve your goal otherwise it will just be a dream

2) Setting unrealistic goals and expectations

Just as not setting a goal can impact your progress, setting unrealistic goals can also. Building muscle is slow and steady; don't believe the ads or fake gurus telling you can gain 50 pounds of muscle in 6 months because it is simply not possible otherwise everyone would be walking around with the bodies they wanted. You can at most, if you're a complete newbie, hope to gain 1 – 2 pounds of quality muscle a month. So don't be deterred if progress is slow, I like to think of it like saving money, you put away a small amount each month but eventually before you look around that small amount has turned into something substantial. Don't let this put you off though because it will be well worth the ordeal when you get there, you will just have to learn to enjoy the process!

3) Not tracking your workouts

How are you supposed to continually make progress if you don't know where you've come from? Every workout should be a battle to beat your last one, whether that's increasing the weight used, doing more reps or more sets you should always endeavour to best yourself. I have yet to meet someone who completely remembers every single variable from his last workout so it's imperative that you keep a logbook. Things you should track are:

- Exercises used
- Weight used
- Sets and Reps done
- Time taken
- Rest periods

4) Not tracking your nutrition

So many skinny guys that I've coached complain that they can't put on weight, they claim, "I eat so much!" But when I actually ask them to keep a daily food log, you can instantly see that they either aren't really eating that much or the foods they eat aren't calorically dense enough. The same usually applies to people looking to lose weight as well. When you think about it logically, how do you expect to build muscle or lose fat without tracking your nutrition? It's like trying to save money without looking at your income. You can't or if you do, it won't be consistent. Just like your workout log, it is vital to your success that you keep a food log as well. Things you should track are:

- Meals
- Calories consumed
- Macronutrient intake e.g. Protein, Carbs, Fats
- Water intake

5) Reliance on supplements

So many people rely on the newest proteins shakes, fat burner pills, pre-workouts etc. What the big supplements companies don't want you to know is that you actually don't need to take anything to build an attractive body; the most anabolic thing you can "take" is food. Do you think the Spartans carried around protein shakes in their sacks? Of course not! The secret is in the name "Supplement". They are meant to supplement your diet; if you haven't got your diet in check then supplements won't do the least bit to help. Supplements are like the cherry on top of an all ready tasty cake. The first thing I would recommend is getting your diet in order before you even think about introducing protein shakes or pre workouts.

6) Consistency

The last point I want to hammer home about is consistency. No training program will ever work for you if you're not consistent. Don't pick and choose when you 'feel like it' or 'had a bad day'; stick to your regime and the rewards will outweigh the hard work.

CHAPTER 5: THE STRENGTH AND MASS PROGRAM GUIDELINES

The Strength and Mass program relies on a very simple set of guidelines that will ensure that you are building muscle and getting stronger week in and week out.

1. **Progressively overload your muscles every workout**
2. **Train in the 4 – 15 rep range**
3. **Do 12 – 16 sets per muscle group**
4. **3 – 4 compound movements per muscle group**
5. **Train each muscle group twice a week.**
6. **Keep a log book!**

Progressively overload your muscles every workout

This is the cornerstone behind every training session and should be used to see if your workouts have been successful.

Train in the 4 – 15 rep range

You will do work within rep ranges of between 4 and 15 on almost every exercise during the program. This will ensure that you hit a variety of muscle fibres. These are the rep ranges that I have found to be the happy medium between building super strength and rock hard muscle consistently.

Do 12 – 16 sets per muscle group

Regardless of the exercises used, you will do 12 – 16 total sets per muscle group. Many strength-based programs simply do not allow enough volume to induce muscle growth and on the other hand, some programs have you pounding out up to 25 sets per muscle group, which is crazy! Not even an adult gorilla could recover from that!

3 – 4 compound movements per muscle group

The Strength and Mass program requires that you use at least 3 compound movements per muscle group. Compound movements allow you to achieve maximum muscle stimulation as they involve more than one muscle group and allow you to use the heaviest amount of weight.

Train each muscle group twice a week.

Training each muscle twice a week ensures enough volume to grow and also allows the muscle to adequately recover and grow. The program is based around different movement patterns - a push/pull/legs split.

Keep a log book!

Finally you must keep a log book otherwise you simply will not know what your goals are for that workout. You must also log your weight every week. Choose a day that best suits you, stick to this day, and always weigh yourself on an empty stomach to get an accurate reading.

And there you have it, stick to these guidelines and you will experience incredible muscle growth and build superhuman strength in the fastest time possible.

Strength and Mass Workout Structure

The Strength and Mass 26 Week program is split into 5 phases. Each phase consists of 5 micro cycles. Micro cycles are a form of training periodization based at the weekly level meaning each week, one of the workout variables will change. For the first week of each cycle, you will perform 3 sets. The second week you will perform 4 sets and the third week you will perform 5 sets. On the fourth week, we will drop the sets back down to 3 but you will increase the weight. Take each set at a time and push yourself to your max, if you need to decrease the weight to stay within the rep ranges then do so!

E.g. Week 1 – 3 x 4 – 6   (75ibs)

   Week 2 - 4 x 4 - 6   (75ibs)

   Week 3 - 5 x 4 – 6   (75ibs)

   Week 4 - 3 x 4 - 6   (80ibs)

Workouts

For each muscle group, you will have two workouts to perform, which you will alternate between. One will be lower in volume but higher in weight; this is your "Strength" based workout and will be targeting myofibrillar hypertrophy. The other will be with much higher reps and volume but with less weight. This is your "Mass" based workout and will be used to target sarcoplasmic hypertrophy. With each workout you must stick between the rep ranges stated. For instance, if an exercise calls for 3 sets of 8 – 10, then you will use a weight that is light enough for you get at least 8 reps but heavy enough that you can do no more than 10 reps. If you can only do 7 reps than the weight is too heavy and vice versa if you can do more than 10 reps than the weight is too light.

An Ideal Split

The split we will be using for the Strength and Mass program *(Push/ Pull / Legs / Rest / Repeat)*. This split is tried and true and allows us to use just enough volume whilst hitting each muscle group every 4 days. If you find that you're not recovering from your workouts, you can always add an extra rest day between your 'Strength' and 'Mass' days.

Example:

Sunday – Push (A)

Monday – Pull (A)

Tuesday – Legs (A)

Wednesday - Rest

Thursday – Push (B)

Friday – Pull (B)

Saturday – Legs (B)

Sunday – Rest

Monday – Push (A)

Beginner split

If you have had less than one year of consistent training, then I would recommend a *Push/Rest/Pull/Rest/Legs/Rest* repeat split or *Push A/Pull A/Legs A/Rest/Rest/Push B/Pull B/Legs B/Rest/Rest/Repeat.*

Example:

Sunday – Push (A)

Monday –Rest

Tuesday – Pull (A)

Wednesday - Rest

Thursday –Legs (A)

Friday – Rest

Saturday – Push (B)

Sunday – Rest

Monday – Pull (B)

Tuesday – Rest

Wednesday – Legs (B)

Deload Weeks

Deload weeks have been integrated into the program to ensure you don't over-train. On deload weeks, you will still train with the same intensity e.g. You will use the same weights and still push yourself, however as the volume of sets will be drastically reduced, it will allow you to fully recover and push beyond your previous boundaries. Some Deload weeks will require you to take a full week off. During these weeks there will be no training whatsoever.

Rest Periods

On 'Strength' days (A) you will rest between 3 – 5 minutes between sets and on 'Mass' days (B) you will rest between 1 – 2 minutes.

Chapter 6: The Strength and Mass warm up protocol

You must warm up every muscle group you are about to train properly before commencing exercise. Training without warming up is a recipe for injury. The point of a warm up is to warm up the muscle that is going to be worked, however many trainees go wrong buy actually fatiguing the muscle. This in turn takes away from your work sets, as most probably you will not be able to use as heavy weights. This method of warming up that I'm about to teach you is one that I have used for years to great effect. It properly warms up the muscles without fatiguing them.

The proper way to warm up

Okay let's take squats for an example. Let's say that you're going to use 300lbs as your weight.

Warm up set 1: 150lbs for 10 reps

The first warm up set is done with roughly half the weight you're going to use for your work sets and should feel very light. It is an opportunity to rehearse and mentally prepare for the movement. Don't go too fast or too slow and focus on increasing the blood flow to the area. Rest for 90 seconds.

Warm up Set 2: Same as Warm up set 1

Warm up Set 3: 200lbs for 5 reps

The third set should be done with roughly 70% of your working weight. It should still feel pretty light. Again don't go too fast or too slow. Rest for 90 seconds

Warm up Set 4: 275 for 1 rep

The fourth and final warm up set should be done with around 80 -90% of your working weight. The purpose here is to prepare the muscle for the heavy weight to come. Rest for 2 minutes before starting your work sets.

Set 1, 2, 3 etc. 300lbs for 4 – 6 reps

These are your work sets; these are the sets that are going to result in muscle growth and strength.

Do I need to warm up again on the next exercise

If the next exercise is the targeting the same muscle group than no.; for instance if you started with squats than went on to the leg press. If you are changing muscle groups, for instance from legs to back, then repeat the same warm up sets above for the next muscle group. The only exception to this would be biceps and triceps as biceps get heavily worked in all pulling movements and triceps get heavily worked in all pushing movements.

CHAPTER 7: THE STRENGTH AND MASS NUTRITION GUIDELINES

This program is all about packing on as much mass as possible, if you want to lose weight than this diet is probably not for you. Your nutrition can make or break the results you get. Because of the volume and intensity of the program, you will need to take in a surplus of calories to adequately repair and grow your muscles.

Calculating your calories

In order to effectively build as much muscle as possible and minimize fat gain, you need to know how many calories to take in each day. Here are some rough guidelines to start from:

Calories needed on Workout Days: 20 calories per pound of bodyweight

Calories needed on Non-Training Days: 18 calories per pound of bodyweight

Once you figure out your calories, it's important to spread them out across 4 – 5 meals throughout the day.

Calculating your Macronutrients split

In case you didn't know, macronutrients = Protein, Fats, Carbohydrates

The macronutrient breakdown has been designed this way as on your training days, you're going to need more energy, which is why there is a higher ratio of carbohydrates. The reason why there is higher protein on your non-training days is because you want to optimally recover.

Training Days

Protein: 30%

Daily Calories needed x 0.3

Carbohydrates: 50%

Daily Calories needed x 0.5

Fats: 20%

Daily Calories needed x 0.2

Non-Training Days

Protein: 40%

Daily Calories needed x 0.4

Carbohydrates: 30%

Daily Calories needed x 0.3

Fats: 30%

Daily Calories needed x 0.3

To work out the amount of grams you need to eat per macronutrient you need first know that:

A gram of protein contains 4 calories

A gram of carbohydrates contains 4 calories

A gram of fat contains 9 calories

Simply divide the amount of calories the macronutrient contains by the calorie requirement.

Here's a calculation of somebody weighing 175 lbs:

175 x 20 = 3500

175 x 18 = 3150

Calories on workout days = 3500

Calories on non-workout days = 3150

Training Days

Daily Calories x 0.3

3500 x 0.3 = 1050 calories needed from protein sources

Daily Calories x 0.5

3500 x 0.5 = 1750 calories needed from carbohydrates

Daily Calories x 0.2

3500 x 0.2 = 700 calories needed from fats

Non-Training Days

Daily Calories x 0.4

3150 x 0.4 = 1260 calories needed from protein sources

Daily Calories x 0.3

3150 x 0.3 = 945 calories needed from carbohydrates

Daily Calories x 0.3

3150 x 0.3 = 945 calories needed from fat

Next in order to work out how many grams are needed per macronutrient just divide the numbers you just calculated above by 4 for protein, 4 for carbs, and 9 for fats

Training Days

1050 Protein calorie requirement / 4 = 262.5 grams

1750 Carbohydrate calorie requirement / 4 = 437.5 grams

700 Fat calorie requirement / 9 = 77.7 grams

Non-Training Days

1260 Protein calorie requirement / 4 = 315 grams

945 Carbohydrate calorie requirement / 4 = 236.2 grams

945 Fat calorie requirement / 9 =105 grams

You want to be gaining about 0.5 – 1 pound a week during the Strength and Mass program. Any more than that and you will be gaining too much fat. If you find you aren't gaining weight, increase your calories by around 100-200 kcals each week until you reach the sweet spot.

Alternatively if you're gaining too much, then you want to reduce your calories by around 100 – 200 each week.

Macronutrient sources

These are the foods you should be eating for the majority of your time on the program. The occasional cheat meal won't harm you but make sure you limit your cheat meals to once or twice a week MAX. For the rest of the time you will choose between these choices!

Your Go to Protein Sources are:

- Chicken

- Turkey

- Cottage cheese

- Whole Eggs

- Egg Whites

- Fish (Any type)

- Beef

- Pork

- Protein Powder

Your Go To Carbohydrates Sources are:

- Sweet potatoes

- Potatoes

- Veggies (Have a least 4 servings of your favourites per day)

- Fruits

- Whole bread

- Brown rice

- Bran cereals

- Whole wheat pasta

- Oats

- Quinoa

- Kidney beans

Your Go To Fat Sources are:

- Egg yolks

- Coconut oil

- Olive oil

- Avocado

- Flax seed oil

- Omega 3 (fish oil capsules)

- Primrose oil

- Canola oil

- Nuts and seeds

- Fatty fish

- Natural nut butter

Water

It is absolutely essential to drink enough water. When you don't get enough, performance can be severely affected. Therefore try to get in about 3 – 4 liters of pure, clean water per day.

CHAPTER 8: SMART SUPPLEMENTATION

Do you need to take supplements to achieve the body you want? Hell No! The key is in the name – supplements. You can build an amazing body just relying on good old fashion food. However supplements can make life more convenient. The supplements below are the only ones I would ever recommend and are ranked in this order.

General Supplements

1) Whey or Casein Protein powder

It can be hard to get in the amount of protein you need from whole foods. This is where protein powder can come in useful. Most protein powders have around 20 – 30 grams of protein per serving which can easily allow you to hit your numbers. Whey protein is fast acting, meaning the body digests it quickly, which makes it perfect for use after a bout of training. Casein protein on the other hand is a slow digesting protein. It can take your body up to 8 hours to fully digest it meaning its great for use when you might have to go without food for a long time or before bedtime to keep you anabolic during the night.

2) Multivitamin

A multivitamin is basically an insurance policy. If you cannot get the necessary vitamins and minerals through your diet than a multivitamin can cover those nutritional gaps.

3) Fish Oils

Fish Oils have been proven to have a number of great health benefits. Fish oils contain "omega 3" fatty acids which cannot be produced by the body and can only be gotten through diet. Fish oils have been shown to reduce inflammation, lower cholesterol, decrease soreness, increase protein synthesis and decrease body fat.

Supplements for performance

4) Creatine Monohydrate (Powder Form)

Creatine is one of the most researched supplements in the world and has shown to have some performance benefits. Benefits include better recovery in-between sets and increased strength.

Chapter 9: Smart Cardio

The Strength and Mass program will require you to do one cardio session per week. The reason for this is it allows you to build muscle without excessive fat gain. Strength and Mass cardio is to be done on one of your rest days. Cardio has three main benefits:

1) Improves endurance
2) Improves your cardiovascular health
3) Burns calories (Great if you're trying to lose body fat)

You can see from these points that cardio is very important for maintaining your overall health however excessive amounts of cardio or the wrong kind of cardio can actually be counter-productive to your muscle building pursuits. If done wrong it can actually cause you to lose muscle mass! How do we maintain our overall health without burning off our hard earned muscle? Enter High intensity interval training.

High intensity interval training (HIIT)

High intensity interval training is essentially where you alternate between periods of high intensity and low intensity. HIIT can be applied to literally anything such as running, cycling on rowing. HIIT has been shown in many studies to be superior to traditional steady state cardio in burning more fat in less time and also "muscle sparing".

Size and Strength Cardio guidelines

- Any machine of your choice e.g. Cycle, Rowing machine etc.
- 30 seconds low intensity + 30 seconds minute high intensity = 1 interval
- 7 to 10 intervals per cardio sessions

Key Points

Always start your cardio sessions with about 2 minutes of low intensity work just to mentally prepare your mind and body for what's to come.

When I say high intensity that means balls to the wall, go to you explode, all out effort for that one minute, nothing should be left on the table. These cardio workouts will make a man out of you very quickly!

After 30 seconds of high intensity, slow done but don't stop. Allow yourself to recover and mentally prepare for the next bout.

CHAPTER 10: THE STRENGTH AND MASS PROGRAM (PHASE 1)

"No citizen has a right to be an amateur in the matter of physical training... what a disgrace it is for a man to grow old without ever seeing the beauty and strength of which his body is capable."
– Socrates

Here we go! This is what you have been waiting for. Make sure you fully understand the guidelines before you start the program. This program is going to demand a lot from you, mentally and physically. There are going to be days when you are going to be sore beyond belief, days when all you will want to do is half – ass it. The difference between winning and losing is simply perseverance. 6 months is a substantial journey and can seem daunting at first. You will be a different person 6 months from now, both mentally but most importantly physically. Take each day at a time, take each set at a time, take each meal at a time and don't give up!

Before you start, you must take your before photos, measurements and starting weight; you'll see a drastic difference in the coming weeks and we'll review your measurements every 10 cycles to ensure progression. Lets begin.

Quick Reminder - Lifting & Rest Days

The split will be using for the Strength and Mass program is the Push/ Pull / Legs / Rest / Repeat. If you have had less than one year of consistent training, or feel like you are not recovering from workout to workout then I would recommend taking two rest days between your 'Strength' and 'Mass' workouts e.g. Push A/Pull A/Legs A/Rest/Rest/Push B/Pull B/Legs B/Rest/Rest/Repeat.

Phase 1

Cycle 1

Push (A) Strength

Bench Press: **3 x 4 – 6**

Incline Bench Press: **3 x 4 – 6**

Seated Barbell overhead shoulder press: **3 x 4 – 6**

Weighted Triceps dip: **3 x 4 - 6**

Pull (A) Strength

Barbell Deadlift: **3 x 4 - 6**

Barbell Bent over row: **3 x 4 - 6**

Weighted Pull-up: **3 x 4-6**

Barbell shrug: **3 x 4-6**

Barbell curl: **3 x 4-6**

Legs (A) Strength

Barbell Squat: **3 x 4 - 6**

Stiff Leg deadlift: **3 x 4-6**

Standing barbell calf raise: **3 x 4-6**

Seated calf raise: **3 x 4 – 6**

Push (B) Size

Dumbbell Bench Press: **3 x 8 – 10**

Incline Dumbbell Flyes: **3 x 12 – 15**

Arnold Press: **3 x 8 – 10**

Dumbbell Lateral Raise: **3 x 12 - 15**

Close grip bench press: **3 x 8 - 10**

Overhead seated Tricep extension: **3 x 8 -10**

Pull (B) Size

Barbell row: **3 x 8-10**

Close grip Lat pull-down: **3 x 8-10**

Cable row: **3 x 8– 10**

EZ Bar curls: **3 x 8- 10**

Cross body Hammer Curls: **3 x 8 - 10**

Legs (B) Size

Barbell Squat : **3 x 8-10**

Leg Press: **3 x 8 - 10**

Leg Curl : **3 x 8 -10**

Leg Extension: **3 x 8-10**

Standing barbell calf raise: **3 x 12-15**

Seated calf raise: **3 x 12 – 15**

Cable crunch: **3 x 10-12**

Hanging Leg Raises: **3 x 10 – 12**

Cycle 2

Push (A) Strength

Bench Press: **4 x 4 – 6**

Incline Bench Press: **4 x 4 – 6**

Seated Barbell overhead shoulder press: **4 x 4 – 6**

Weighted Triceps dip: **4 x 4 - 6**

Pull (A) Strength

Barbell Deadlift: **4 x 4 - 6**

Barbell Bent over row: **4 x 4 - 6**

Weighted Pull-up: **4 x 4-6**

Barbell shrug: **4 x 4-6**

Barbell curl: **4 x 4-6**

Legs (A) Strength

Barbell Squat: **4 x 4 - 6**

Stiff Leg deadlift: **4 x 4-6**

Standing barbell calf raise: **4 x 4-6**

Seated calf raise: **4 x 4 – 6**

Push (B) Size

Dumbbell Bench Press: **4 x 8 – 10**

Incline Dumbbell Flyes: **4 x 12 – 15**

Arnold Press: **4 x 8 – 10**

Dumbbell Lateral Raise: **4 x 12 - 15**

Close grip bench press: **4 x 8 - 10**

Overhead seated Tricep extension: **4 x 8 -10**

Pull (B) Size

Barbell row: **4 x 8-10**

Close grip Lat pull-down: **4 x 8-10**

Cable row: **4 x 8– 10**

EZ Bar curls: **4 x 8- 10**

Cross body Hammer Curls: **4 x 8 - 10**

Legs (B) Size

Barbell Squat **: 4 x 8-10**

Leg Press: **4 x 8 - 10**

Leg Curl : **4 x 8 -10**

Leg Extension: **4 x 8-10**

Standing barbell calf raise: **4 x 12-15**

Seated calf raise: **4 x 12 – 15**

Cable crunch: **4 x 10-12**

Hanging Leg Raises: **4 x 10 – 12**

Cycle 3

Push (A) Strength

Bench Press: **5 x 4 – 6**

Incline Bench Press: **5 x 4 – 6**

Seated Barbell overhead shoulder press: **5 x 4 – 6**

Weighted Triceps dip: **5 x 4 - 6**

Pull (A) Strength

Barbell Deadlift: **5 x 4 - 6**

Barbell Bent over row: **5 x 4 - 6**

Weighted Pull up: **5 x 4-6**

Barbell shrug: **5 x 4-6**

Barbell curl: **5 x 4-6**

Legs (A) Strength

Barbell Squat: **5 x 4 - 6**

Stiff Leg deadlift: **5 x 4-6**

Standing barbell calf raise: **5 x 4-6**

Seated calf raise: **5 x 4 – 6**

Push (B) Size

Dumbbell Bench Press: **5 x 8 – 10**

Incline Dumbbell Press: **5 x 8 – 10**

Incline Dumbbell Flyes: **5 x 12 – 15**

Arnold Press: **5 x 8 – 10**

Upright Row: **5 x 8 - 10**

Dumbbell Lateral Raise: **5 x 12 - 15**

Close grip bench press: **5 x 8 - 10**

Overhead seated Tricep extension: **5 x 8 -10**

Pull (B) Size

Barbell row: **5 x 8-10**

Close grip Lat pull-down: **5 x 8-10**

Cable row: **5 x 8– 10**

EZ Bar curls: **5 x 8- 10**

Cross body Hammer Curls: **5 x 8 – 10**

Legs (B) Size

Barbell Squat **: 5 x 8-10**

Leg Press: **5 x 8 - 10**

Leg Curl : **5 x 8 -10**

Leg Extension: **5 x 8-10**

Standing barbell calf raise: **5 x 12-15**

Seated calf raise: **5 x 12 – 15**

Cable crunch: **5 x 10-12**

Hanging Leg Raises: **5 x 10 – 12**

Cycle 4

(Increase the weight on all exercises by 5-10%)

Push (A) Strength

Bench Press: **3 x 4 – 6**

Incline Bench Press: **3 x 4 – 6**

Seated Barbell overhead shoulder press: **3 x 4 – 6**

Weighted Triceps dip: **3 x 4 - 6**

Pull (A) Strength

Barbell Deadlift: **3 x 4 - 6**

Barbell Bent over row: **3 x 4 - 6**

Weighted Pull-up: **3 x 4-6**

Barbell shrug: **3 x 4-6**

Barbell curl: **3 x 4-6**

Legs (A) Strength

Barbell Squat: **3 x 4 - 6**

Stiff Leg deadlift: **3 x 4-6**

Standing barbell calf raise: **3 x 4-6**

Seated calf raise: **3 x 4 – 6**

Push (B) Size

Dumbbell Bench Press: **3 x 8 – 10**

Incline Dumbbell Press: **3 x 8 – 10**

Incline Dumbbell Flyes: **3 x 12 – 15**

Arnold Press: **3 x 8 – 10**

Upright Row: **3 x 8 - 10**

Dumbbell Lateral Raise: **3 x 12 - 15**

Close grip bench press: **3 x 8 - 10**

Overhead seated Tricep extension: **3 x 8 -10**

Pull (B) Size

Barbell row: **3 x 8-10**

Close grip Lat pull-down: **3 x 8-10**

Cable row: **3 x 8– 10**

EZ Bar curls: **3 x 8- 10**

Cross body Hammer Curls: **5 x 8 - 10**

Legs (B) Size

Barbell Squat: **3 x 8-10**

Leg Press: **3 x 8 - 10**

Leg Curl: **3 x 8 -10**

Leg Extension: **3 x 8-10**

Standing barbell calf raise: **3 x 12-15**

Seated calf raise: **3 x 12 – 15**

Cable crunch: **3 x 10-12**

Hanging Leg Raises: **3 x 10 – 12**

Cycle 5 (Deload)

Push (A) Strength

Bench Press: **1 x 4 – 6**

Incline Bench Press: **1 x 4 – 6**

Seated Barbell overhead shoulder press: **1 x 4 – 6**

Weighted Triceps dip: **1 x 4 - 6**

Pull (A) Strength

Barbell Deadlift: **1 x 4 - 6**

Barbell Bent over row: **1 x 4 - 6**

Weighted Pull-up: **1 x 4-6**

Barbell shrug: **1 x 4-6**

Barbell curl: **1 x 4-6**

Legs (A) Strength

Barbell Squat: **1 x 4 - 6**

Stiff Leg deadlift: **1 x 4-6**

Standing barbell calf raise: **1 x 4-6**

Seated calf raise: **1 x 4 – 6**

Push (B) Size

Dumbbell Bench Press: **1 x 8 – 10**

Incline Dumbbell Press: **1 x 8 – 10**

Incline Dumbbell Flyes: **1 x 12 – 15**

Arnold Press: **1 x 8 – 10**

Upright Row: **1 x 8 - 10**

Dumbbell Lateral Raise: **1 x 12 - 15**

Close grip bench press: **1 x 8 - 10**

Overhead seated Tricep extension: **1 x 8 -10**

Pull (B) Size

Barbell row: **1 x 8-10**

Close grip Lat pull-down: **1 x 8-10**

Cable row: **1 x 8– 10**

EZ Bar curls: **1 x 8- 10**

Cross body Hammer Curls: **1 x 8 - 10**

Legs (B) Size

Barbell Squat**: 1 x 8-10**

Leg Press: **1 x 8 - 10**

Leg Curl: **1 x 8 -10**

Leg Extension: **1 x 8-10**

Standing barbell calf raise: **1 x 12-15**

Seated calf raise**: 1 x 12 – 15**

Cable crunch: **1 x 10-12**

Hanging Leg Raises: **1 x 10 – 12**

Cycle 6

Push (A) Strength

Incline Dumbbell Press: **3 x 3 – 5**

Dumbbell Bench Press: **3 x 3 – 5**

Standing Barbell overhead shoulder press: **3 x 3 – 5**

Close grip bench press: **3 x 4 - 6**

Pull (A) Strength

Barbell Bent over row: **3 x 3 - 5**

Wide grip Weighted Pull-up: **3 x 3 - 5**

Barbell shrug: **3 x 3-5**

Dumbbell curl: **3 x 4-6**

Legs (A) Strength

Front Squat: **3 x 3 - 5**

Stiff leg deadlift: **3 x 3 - 5**

Seated calf raise: **3 x 4 – 6**

Standing barbell calf raise: **3 x 4-6**

Push (B) Size

Bench Press: **3 x 6 – 8**

Incline Bench Press: **3 x 8 – 10**

Cable Flyes: **3 x 12 – 15**

Seated dumbbell Shoulder Press: **3 x 6– 8**

Smith machine Upright Row: **3 x 8 - 10**

Cable Lateral Raise: **3 x 12 - 15**

Weighted dip **3 x 6 - 8**

Tricep pushdown: **3 x 8 -10**

Pull (B) Size

T-Bar row: **3 x 6-8**

Wide grip Lat pull-down: **3 x 8-10**

Dumbbell row: **3 x 12– 15**

Barbell curls: **3 x 6- 8**

Incline dumbbell curl: **3 x 8 - 10**

Legs (B) Size

Hack Squat: **3 x 6-8**

Leg Press: **3 x 8 - 10**

Leg Curl: **3 x 8 -10**

Leg Extension: **3 x 12-15**

Standing barbell calf raise: **3 x 12-15**

Seated calf raise: **3 x 12 – 15**

Cable crunch: **3 x 10-12**

Hanging Leg Raises: **3 x 10 – 12**

Cycle 7

Push (A) Strength

Incline Dumbbell Press: **4 x 3– 5**

Dumbbell Bench Press: **4 x 3– 5**

Standing Barbell overhead shoulder press: **4 x 3 – 5**

Close grip bench press: **4 x 4 - 6**

Pull (A) Strength

Barbell Bent over row: **4 x 3 - 5**

Wide grip Weighted Pull-up: **4 x 3-5**

Barbell shrug: **4 x 3-5**

Dumbbell curl: **4 x 4-6**

Legs (A) Strength

Front Squat: **4 x 3 - 5**

Stiff leg deadlift: **4 x 3 -5**

Seated calf raise: **4 x 4 – 6**

Standing barbell calf raise: **4 x 4-6**

Push (B) Size

Bench Press: **4 x 6 – 8**

Incline Bench Press: **4 x 8 – 10**

Cable Flyes: **4 x 12 – 15**

Seated dumbbell Shoulder Press: **4 x 6 – 8**

Smith machine Upright Row: **4 x 8 - 10**

Cable Lateral Raise: **4 x 12 - 15**

Weighted dip **4 x 6 - 8**

Tricep pushdown: **4 x 8 -10**

Pull (B) Size

T-Bar row: **4 x 6-8**

Wide grip Lat pull-down: **4 x 8-10**

Dumbbell row: **4 x 12– 15**

Barbell curls: **4 x 6- 8**

Incline dumbbell curl: **4 x 8 – 10**

Legs (B) Size

Hack Squat: **4 x 6-8**

Leg Press: **4 x 8 - 10**

Leg Curl : **4 x 8 -10**

Leg Extension: **4 x 12-15**

Standing barbell calf raise: **4 x 12-15**

Seated calf raise: **4 x 12 – 15**

Cable crunch: **4 x 10-12**

Hanging Leg Raises: **4 x 10 – 12**

Cycle 8

Push (A) Strength

Incline Dumbbell Press: **5 x 3 -5**

Dumbbell Bench Press: **5 x 3 –5**

Standing Barbell overhead shoulder press: **5 x 3 – 5**

Close grip bench press: **5 x 4 - 6**

Pull (A) Strength

Barbell Bent over row: **5 x 3 - 5**

Wide grip Weighted Pull-up: **5 x 3-5**

Barbell shrug: **5 x 3-5**

Dumbbell curl: **5 x 4-6**

Legs (A) Strength

Front Squat: **5 x 3-5**

Stiff leg deadlift: **5 x 3-5**

Seated calf raise: **5 x 4 – 6**

Standing barbell calf raise: **5 x 4-6**

Push (B) Size

Bench Press: **5 x 6 – 8**

Incline Bench Press: **5 x 8 – 10**

Cable Flyes: **5 x 12 – 15**

Seated dumbbell Shoulder Press: **5 x 6– 8**

Smith machine Upright Row: **5 x 8 - 10**

Cable Lateral Raise: **5 x 12 - 15**

Weighted dip **5 x 6 - 8**

Tricep pushdown: **4 x 8 -10**

Pull (B) Size

T-Bar row: **5 x 6-8**

Wide grip Lat pull-down: **5 x 8-10**

Dumbbell row: **5 x 12– 15**

Barbell curls: **5 x 6- 8**

Incline dumbbell curl: **5 x 8 - 10**

Legs (B) Size

Hack Squat **: 5 x 6-8**

Leg Press: **5 x 8 - 10**

Leg Curl : **5 x 8 -10**

Leg Extension: **5 x 12-15**

Standing barbell calf raise: **5 x 12-15**

Seated calf raise**: 5 x 12 – 15**

Cable crunch: **5 x 10-12**

Hanging Leg Raises: **5 x 10 – 12**

Cycle 9

(Increase the weight on all exercises by 5-10%)

Push (A) Strength

Incline Dumbbell Press: **3 x 3-5**

Dumbbell Bench Press: **3 x 3 – 5**

Standing Barbell overhead shoulder press: **3 x 3 – 5**

Close grip bench press: **3 x 4 - 6**

Pull (A) Strength

Barbell Bent over row: **3 x 3 - 5**

Wide grip Weighted Pull-up: **3 x 3-5**

Barbell shrug: **3 x 3-5**

Dumbbell curl: **3 x 4-6**

Legs (A) Strength

Front Squat: **3 x 3-5**

Stiff leg deadlift: **3 x 3-5**

Seated calf raise: **3 x 4-6**

Standing barbell calf raise: **3 x 4-6**

Push (B) Size

Bench Press: **3 x 6 – 8**

Incline Bench Press: **3 x 8 – 10**

Cable Flyes: **3 x 12 – 15**

Seated dumbbell Shoulder Press: **3 x 8 – 10**

Smith machine Upright Row: **3 x 8 - 10**

Cable Lateral Raise: **3 x 12 - 15**

Weighted dip **3 x 6 - 8**

Tricep pushdown: **3 x 8 -10**

Pull (B) Size

T-Bar row: **3 x 6-8**

Wide grip Lat pull-down: **3 x 8-10**

Dumbbell row: **3 x 8– 10**

Barbell curls: **3 x 8- 10**

Incline dumbbell curl: **3 x 8 - 10**

Legs (B) Size

Hack Squat: **3 x 6-8**

Leg Press: **3 x 8 - 10**

Leg Curl: **3 x 8 -10**

Leg Extension: **3 x 12-15**

Standing barbell calf raise: **3 x 12-15**

Seated calf raise: **3 x 12 – 15**

Cable crunch: **3 x 10-12**

Hanging Leg Raises: **3 x 10 – 12**

Cycle 10 (Deload)

Push (A) Strength

Incline Dumbbell Press: **1 x 3-5**

Dumbbell Bench Press: **1 x 3–5**

Standing Barbell overhead shoulder press: **1 x 3-5**

Close grip bench press: **1 x 4 - 6**

Pull (A) Strength

Barbell Bent over row: **1 x 3-5**

Wide grip Weighted Pull-up: **1 x 3-5**

Barbell shrug: **1 x 3-5**

Dumbbell curl: **1 x 4-6**

Legs (A) Strength

Front Squat: **1 x 3 - 5**

Stiff leg deadlift: **1 x 3-5**

Seated calf raise: **1 x 3 – 5**

Standing barbell calf raise: **1 x 4-6**

Push (B) Size

Bench Press: **1 x 6 – 8**

Incline Bench Press: **1 x 8 – 10**

Cable Flyes: **1 x 12 – 15**

Seated dumbbell Shoulder Press: **1 x 6– 8**

Smith machine Upright Row: **1 x 8 - 10**

Cable Lateral Raise: **1 x 12 - 15**

Weighted dip **1 x 6-8**

Tricep pushdown: **1 x 8 -10**

Pull (B) Size

T-Bar row: **1 x 6-8**

Wide grip Lat pull-down: **1 x 8-10**

Dumbbell row: **1 x 12– 15**

Barbell curls: **1 x 6- 8**

Incline dumbbell curl: **1 x 8 - 10**

Legs (B) Size

Hack Squat: **1 x 6-8**

Leg Press: **1 x 8 - 10**

Leg Curl: **1 x 8 -10**

Leg Extension: **1 x 12-15**

Standing barbell calf raise: **1 x 12-15**

Seated calf raise: **1 x 12 – 15**

Cable crunch: **1 x 10-12**

Hanging Leg Raises: **1 x 10 - 12**

Well done on completing the first 10 cycles!

Time to take some more measurements and progress pictures. By now you should be considerably stronger than when you first started, and will have started to notice changes in your physique. Keep up the good work!

(PHASE 3)

Cycle 11

Push (A) Strength

Bench Press: **4 x 4 – 6**

Incline Bench Press: **3 x 4 – 6**

Seated Barbell overhead shoulder press: **4 x 4 – 6**

Weighted Triceps dip: **3 x 4 - 6**

Pull (A) Strength

Barbell Deadlift: **4 x 4 - 6**

Barbell Bent over row: **3 x 4 - 6**

Weighted Pull-up: **4 x 4-6**

Barbell shrug: **3 x 4-6**

Barbell curl: **4 x 4-6**

Legs (A) Strength

Barbell Squat: **4 x 4 - 6**

Stiff Leg deadlift: **3 x 4-6**

Standing barbell calf raise: **4 x 4-6**

Seated calf raise: **3 x 4 – 6**

Push (B) Size

Dumbbell Bench Press: **4 x 8 – 10**

Incline Dumbbell Flyes: **3 x 12 – 15**

Arnold Press: **4 x 8 – 10**

Dumbbell Lateral Raise: **3 x 12 - 15**

Close grip bench press: **4 x 8 - 10**

Overhead seated Tricep extension: **3 x 8 -10**

Pull (B) Size

Barbell row: **4 x 8-10**

Close grip Lat pull-down: **3 x 8-10**

Cable row: **3 x 8– 10**

EZ Bar curls: **4 x 8- 10**

Cross body Hammer Curls: **3 x 8 - 10**

Legs (B) Size

Barbell Squat: **4 x 8-10**

Leg Press: **3 x 8 - 10**

Leg Curl: **3 x 8 -10**

Leg Extension: **3 x 8-10**

Standing barbell calf raise: **4 x 12-15**

Seated calf raise: **3 x 12 – 15**

Cable crunch: **4 x 10-12**

Hanging Leg Raises: **3 x 10 - 12**

Cycle 12

Push (A) Strength

Bench Press: **5 x 4 – 6**

Incline Bench Press: **4 x 4 – 6**

Seated Barbell overhead shoulder press: **5 x 4 – 6**

Weighted Triceps dip: **4 x 4 - 6**

Pull (A) Strength

Barbell Deadlift: **5 x 4 - 6**

Barbell Bent over row: **4 x 4 - 6**

Weighted Pull-up: **5 x 4-6**

Barbell shrug: **4 x 4-6**

Barbell curl: **5 x 4-6**

Legs (A) Strength

Barbell Squat: **5 x 4 - 6**

Stiff Leg deadlift: **4 x 4-6**

Standing barbell calf raise: **5 x 4-6**

Seated calf raise: **4 x 4 – 6**

Push (B) Size

Dumbbell Bench Press: **5 x 8 – 10**

Incline Dumbbell Flyes: **4 x 12 – 15**

Arnold Press: **5 x 8 – 10**

Dumbbell Lateral Raise: **4 x 12 - 15**

Close grip bench press: **5 x 8 - 10**

Overhead seated Tricep extension: **4 x 8 -10**

Pull (B) Size

Barbell row: **5 x 8-10**

Close grip Lat pull-down: **4 x 8-10**

Cable row: **4 x 8– 10**

EZ Bar curls: **5 x 8- 10**

Cross body Hammer Curls: **4 x 8 - 10**

Legs (B) Size

Barbell Squat: **5 x 8-10**

Leg Press: **4 x 8 - 10**

Leg Curl: **4 x 8 -10**

Leg Extension: **4 x 8-10**

Standing barbell calf raise: **5 x 12-15**

Seated calf raise: **4 x 12 – 15**

Cable crunch: **5 x 10-12**

Hanging Leg Raises: **4 x 10 - 12**

Cycle 13

Push (A) Strength

Bench Press: **6 x 4 – 6**

Incline Bench Press: **5 x 4 – 6**

Seated Barbell overhead shoulder press: **6 x 4 – 6**

Weighted Triceps dip: **5 x 4 - 6**

Pull (A) Strength

Barbell Deadlift: **6 x 4 - 6**

Barbell Bent over row: **5 x 4 - 6**

Weighted Pull up: **6 x 4-6**

Barbell shrug: **5 x 4-6**

Barbell curl: **6 x 4-6**

Legs (A) Strength

Barbell Squat: **6 x 4 - 6**

Stiff Leg deadlift: **5 x 4-6**

Standing barbell calf raise: **6 x 4-6**

Seated calf raise: **5 x 4 – 6**

Push (B) Size

Dumbbell Bench Press: **6 x 8 – 10**

Incline Dumbbell Flyes: **5 x 12 – 15**

Arnold Press: **6 x 8 – 10**

Dumbbell Lateral Raise: **5 x 12 - 15**

Close grip bench press: **6 x 8 - 10**

Overhead seated Tricep extension: **5 x 8 -10**

Pull (B) Size

Barbell row: **6 x 8-10**

Close grip Lat pull-down: **5 x 8-10**

Cable row: **5 x 8– 10**

EZ Bar curls: **6 x 8- 10**

Cross body Hammer Curls: **5 x 8 - 10**

Legs (B) Size

Barbell Squat: **6 x 8-10**

Leg Press: **5 x 8 - 10**

Leg Curl: **5 x 8 -10**

Leg Extension: **5 x 8-10**

Standing barbell calf raise: **6 x 12-15**

Seated calf raise: **5 x 12 – 15**

Cable crunch: **6 x 10-12**

Hanging Leg Raises: **5 x 10 – 12**

Cycle 14

(Increase the weight on all exercises by 5-10%)

Push (A) Strength

Bench Press: **4 x 4 – 6**

Incline Bench Press: **3 x 4 – 6**

Seated Barbell overhead shoulder press: **4 x 4 – 6**

Weighted Triceps dip: **3 x 4 - 6**

Pull (A) Strength

Barbell Deadlift: **4 x 4 - 6**

Barbell Bent over row: **3 x 4 - 6**

Weighted Pullup: **4 x 4-6**

Barbell shrug: **3 x 4-6**

Barbell curl: **4 x 4-6**

Legs (A) Strength

Barbell Squat: **4 x 4 - 6**

Stiff Leg deadlift: **3 x 4-6**

Standing barbell calf raise: **4 x 4-6**

Seated calf raise: **4 x 4 – 6**

Push (B) Size

Dumbbell Bench Press: **4 x 8 – 10**

Incline Dumbbell Press: **3 x 8 – 10**

Incline Dumbbell Flyes: **3 x 12 – 15**

Arnold Press: **3 x 8 – 10**

Upright Row: **3 x 8 - 10**

Dumbbell Lateral Raise: **3 x 12 - 15**

Close grip bench press: **3 x 8 - 10**

Overhead seated Tricep extension: **3 x 8 -10**

Pull (B) Size

Barbell row: **4 x 8-10**

Close grip Lat pull-down: **3 x 8-10**

Cable row: **3 x 8– 10**

EZ Bar curls: **4 x 8- 10**

Cross body Hammer Curls: **3 x 8 - 10**

Legs (B) Size

Barbell Squat**: 3 x 8-10**

Leg Press: **3 x 8 - 10**

Leg Curl: **3 x 8 -10**

Leg Extension: **3 x 8-10**

Standing barbell calf raise: **3 x 12-15**

Seated calf raise: **3 x 12 – 15**

Cable crunch: **3 x 10-12**

Hanging Leg Raises: **3 x 10 - 12**

Cycle 15 (Deload)

Week Off

You've been pounding the weights for a while now. This deload, you will take a full week off from the gym to let you body fully recover. No weight training whatsoever, however don't use this as a excuse to let your nutrition go down hill. Enjoy this week off - you've earned it.

(Phase 4)

Cycle 16

Push (A) Strength

Bench Press: **3 x 4 – 6**

Incline Dumbbell Bench Press: **3 x 4 – 6**

Standing Barbell overhead shoulder press: **3 x 4 – 6**

Triceps pushdown: **3 x 4 - 6**

Pull (A) Strength

T-Bar Row: **3 x 4 - 6**

Weighted Pull-up: **3 x 4-6**

Dumbbell shrug: **3 x 4-6**

Dumbbell curl: **3 x 4-6**

Legs (A) Strength

Front Squat: **3 x 4 - 6**

Sumo deadlift: **3 x 4-6**

Standing barbell calf raise: **3 x 4-6**

Seated calf raise: **3 x 4 – 6**

Push (B) Size

Dumbbell Bench Press: **3 x 10-12**

Incline Dumbbell Press: **3 x 10– 12**

Shoulder Dumbbell Press: **3 x 10–12**

Dumbbell Lateral Raise: **3 x 12 - 15**

Tricep pushdown: **3 x 12 - 15**

Overhead seated Tricep extension: **3 x 12 -15**

Pull (B) Size

Dumbbell row: **3 x 12-15**

Wide grip Lat pull-down: **3 x 12-15**

Cable row: **3 x 12– 15**

Barbell curls: **3 x 12- 15**

Reverse grip Barbell Curls: **3 x 12 - 15**

Legs (B) Size

Barbell Squat: **3 x 12-15**

Leg Press: **3 x 12 - 15**

Leg Curl: **3 x 12 -15**

Leg Extension: **3 x 12-15**

Standing barbell calf raise: **3 x 12-15**

Seated calf raise: **3 x 12 – 15**

Cable crunch: **3 x 10-12**

Hanging Leg Raises: **3 x 10 – 12**

Cycle 17

Push (A) Strength

Bench Press: **4 x 4 – 6**

Incline Dumbbell Press: **4 x 4 – 6**

Standing Barbell overhead shoulder press: **4 x 4 – 6**

Triceps Pushdown: **4 x 4 – 6**

Pull (A) Strength

T-Bar row: **4 x 4 - 6**

Weighted Pull-up: **4 x 4-6**

Dumbbell shrug: **4 x 4-6**

Dumbbell curl: **4 x 4-6**

Legs (A) Strength

Front Squat: **4 x 4 - 6**

Sumo deadlift: **4 x 4-6**

Standing barbell calf raise: **4 x 4-6**

Seated calf raise: **4 x 4 – 6**

Push (B) Size

Dumbbell Bench Press: **4 x 12– 15**

Incline Dumbbell Press: **4 x 12 – 15**

Incline Dumbbell Flyes: **4 x 12 – 15**

Dumbbell Shoulder Press: **4 x 12 – 15**

Dumbbell Lateral Raise: **4 x 12 - 15**

Tricep pushdown: **4 x 12 - 15**

Overhead seated Tricep extension: **4 x 12 -15**

Pull (B) Size

Dumbbell row: **4 x 12-15**

Wide grip Lat pull-down: **4 x 12-15**

Cable row: **4 x 12–15**

Barbell curls: **4 x 12-15**

Reverse Grip Barbell Curls: **4 x 8 - 10**

Legs (B) Size

Barbell Squat: **4 x 12-15**

Leg Press: **4 x 12 - 15**

Leg Curl: **4 x 12 -15**

Leg Extension: **4 x 12-15**

Standing barbell calf raise: **4 x 12-15**

Seated calf raise: **4 x 12 – 15**

Cable crunch: **4 x 10-12**

Hanging Leg Raises: **4 x 10 - 12**

Cycle 18

Push (A) Strength

Bench Press: **5 x 4 – 6**

Incline Dumbbell Bench Press: **5 x 4 – 6**

Standing Barbell overhead shoulder press: **5 x 4 – 6**

Tricep pushdown: **5 x 4 - 6**

Pull (A) Strength

T-Bar row: **5 x 4 - 6**

Weighted Pull-up: **5 x 4-6**

Dumbbell shrug: **5 x 4-6**

Dumbbell curl: **5 x 4-6**

Legs (A) Strength

Front Squat: **5 x 4 - 6**

Sumo deadlift: **5 x 4-6**

Standing barbell calf raise: **5 x 4-6**

Seated calf raise: **5 x 4 – 6**

Push (B) Size

Dumbbell Bench Press: **5 x 12 – 15**

Incline Dumbbell Press: **5 x 12 – 15**

Shoulder Dumbbell Press: **5 x 12– 15**

Dumbbell Lateral Raise: **5 x 12 - 15**

Tricep pushdown: **5 x 12 - 15**

Overhead seated Tricep extension: **5 x 12 -15**

Pull (B) Size

Dumbbell row: **5 x 12-15**

Wide grip Lat pull-down: **5 x 12-15**

Cable row: **5 x 12– 15**

Barbell Curls: **5 x 12- 15**

Cross body Hammer Curls: **5 x 12 - 15**

Legs (B) Size

Barbell Squat: **5 x 12-15**

Leg Press: **5 x 12 - 15**

Leg Curl: **5 x 12 -15**

Leg Extension: **5 x 12-15**

Standing barbell calf raise: **5 x 12-15**

Seated calf raise: **5 x 12 – 15**

Cable crunch: **5 x 10-12**

Hanging Leg Raises: **5 x 10 - 12**

Cycle 19

(Increase the weight on all exercises by 5-10%)

Push (A) Strength

Bench Press: **3 x 4 – 6**

Incline Dumbbell Bench Press: **3 x 4 – 6**

Standing Barbell overhead shoulder press: **5 x 4 – 6**

Triceps pushdown: **3 x 4 - 6**

Pull (A) Strength

T-Bar row: **3 x 4 - 6**

Weighted Pull-up: **3 x 4-6**

Dumbbell shrug: **3 x 4-6**

Dumbbell curl: **3 x 4-6**

Legs (A) Strength

Front Squat: **3 x 4 - 6**

Sumo deadlift: **3 x 4-6**

Standing barbell calf raise: **3 x 4-6**

Seated calf raise: **3 x 4 – 6**

Push (B) Size

Dumbbell Bench Press: **3 x 12 – 15**

Incline Dumbbell Press: **3 x 12 – 15**

Arnold Press: **3 x 12– 15**

Dumbbell Lateral Raise: **3 x 12 - 15**

Tricep pushdown: **3 x 12- 15**

Overhead seated Tricep extension: **3 x 12 -15**

Pull (B) Size

Dumbbell row: **3 x 12-15**

Wide-grip Lat pull-down: **3 x 12-15**

Cable row: **3 x 8– 10**

Barbell curl: **3 x 12- 15**

Reverse grip barbell Curls: **5 x 12- 15**

Legs (B) Size

Barbell Squat: **3 x 12-15**

Leg Press: **3 x 12 - 15**

Leg Curl: **3 x 12-15**

Leg Extension: **3 x 12-15**

Standing barbell calf raise: **3 x 12-15**

Seated calf raise: **3 x 12 – 15**

Cable crunch: **3 x 10-12**

Hanging Leg Raises: **3 x 10 - 12**

Cycle 20 (Deload)

Push (A) Strength

Bench Press: **1 x 4 – 6**

Incline Dumbbell Bench Press: **1 x 4 – 6**

Standing Barbell overhead shoulder press: **1 x 4 – 6**

Tricep pushdown: **1 x 4 - 6**

Pull (A) Strength

T-Bar row: **1 x 4 - 6**

Weighted Pull-up: **1 x 4-6**

Dumbbell shrug: **1 x 4-6**

Dumbbell curl: **1 x 4-6**

Legs (A) Strength

Front Squat: **1 x 4 - 6**

Sumo deadlift: **1 x 4-6**

Standing barbell calf raise: **1 x 4-6**

Seated calf raise: **1 x 4 – 6**

Push (B) Size

Dumbbell Bench Press: **1 x 12 – 15**

Incline Dumbbell Press: **1 x 12– 15**

Incline Dumbbell Flyes: **1 x 12 – 15**

Shoulder Dumbbell Press: **1 x 12 – 15**

Dumbbell Lateral Raise: **1 x 12 - 15**

Tricep pushdown: **1 x 12 - 15**

Overhead seated Tricep extension: **1 x 12 -15**

Pull (B) Size

Dumbbell row: **1 x 12-15**

Wide Grip Lat pull-down: **1 x 12-15**

Cable row: **1 x 12– 15**

Barbell curl: **1 x 12- 15**

Reverse Grip Barbell curls: **1 x 8 – 10**

Legs (B) Size

Barbell Squat: **1 x 12-15**

Leg Press: **1 x 12 - 15**

Leg Curl: **1 x 12 -15**

Leg Extension: **1 x 12-15**

Standing barbell calf raise: **1 x 12-15**

Seated calf raise: **1 x 12 – 15**

Cable crunch: **1 x 10-12**

Hanging Leg Raises: **1 x 10 - 12**

Another 10 cycles have passed and a real physique is starting to take shape. Time to take your measurements!

Every workout so far has built on the last and your strength and mass should be going through the roof! Be prepared for Friends and Co – Workers to complement you. Phase 5 is the final part of the Strength and Mass program, so remember to give it your all.

(PHASE 5)

Cycle 21

Push (A) Strength

Incline Dumbbell Press: **3 x 4 – 6**

Dumbbell Bench Press: **3 x 4 – 6**

Standing Barbell overhead shoulder press: **3 x 4 – 6**

Close grip bench press: **3 x 4 - 6**

Pull (A) Strength

Barbell Bent over row: **3 x 4 - 6**

Wide grip Weighted Pull-up: **3 x 4-6**

Barbell shrug: **3 x 4-6**

Dumbbell curl: **3 x 4-6**

Legs (A) Strength

Front Squat: **3 x 4 - 6**

Stiff leg deadlift: **3 x 4-6**

Seated calf raise: **3 x 4 – 6**

Standing barbell calf raise: **3 x 4-6**

Push (B) Size

Bench Press: **3 x 6 – 8**

Incline Bench Press: **3 x 8 – 10**

Cable Flyes: **3 x 12 – 15**

Seated dumbbell Shoulder Press: **3 x 8 – 10**

Smith machine Upright Row: **3 x 8 - 10**

Cable Lateral Raise: **3 x 12 - 15**

Weighted **3 x 8 - 10**

Tricep pushdown: **3 x 8 -10**

Pull (B) Size

T-Bar row: **3 x 6-8**

Wide grip Lat pull-down: **3 x 8-10**

Dumbbell row: **3 x 8– 10**

Barbell curls: **3 x 8- 10**

Incline dumbbell curl: **3 x 8 - 10**

Legs (B) Size

Hack Squat: **3 x 6-8**

Leg Press: **3 x 8 - 10**

Leg Curl: **3 x 8 -10**

Leg Extension: **3 x 8-10**

Standing barbell calf raise: **3 x 12-15**

Seated calf raise: **3 x 12 – 15**

Cable crunch: **3 x 10-12**

Hanging Leg Raises: **3 x 10 - 12**

Cycle 22

Push (A) Strength

Incline Dumbbell Press: **4 x 4 – 6**

Dumbbell Bench Press: **4 x 4 – 6**

Standing Barbell overhead shoulder press: **4 x 4 – 6**

Close grip bench press: **4 x 4 - 6**

Pull (A) Strength

Barbell Bent over row: **4 x 4 - 6**

Wide grip Weighted Pull-up: **4 x 4-6**

Barbell shrug: **4 x 4-6**

Dumbbell curl: **4 x 4-6**

Legs (A) Strength

Front Squat: **4 x 4 - 6**

Stiff leg deadlift: **4 x 4-6**

Seated calf raise: **4 x 4 – 6**

Standing barbell calf raise: **4 x 4-6**

Push (B) Size

Bench Press: **4 x 6 – 8**

Incline Bench Press: **4 x 8 – 10**

Cable Flyes: **4 x 12 – 15**

Seated dumbbell Shoulder Press: **4 x 8 – 10**

Smith machine Upright Row: **4 x 8 - 10**

Cable Lateral Raise: **4 x 12 - 15**

Weighted dip **4 x 8 - 10**

Tricep pushdown: **4 x 8 -10**

Pull (B) Size

T-Bar row: **4 x 6-8**

Wide grip Lat pull-down: **4 x 8-10**

Dumbbell row: **4 x 8– 10**

Barbell curls: **4 x 8- 10**

Incline dumbbell curl: **4 x 8 - 10**

Legs (B) Size

Hack Squat: **4 x 6-8**

Leg Press: **4 x 8 - 10**

Leg Curl : **4 x 8 -10**

Leg Extension: **4 x 8-10**

Standing barbell calf raise: **4 x 12-15**

Seated calf raise: **4 x 12 – 15**

Cable crunch: **4 x 10-12**

Hanging Leg Raises: **4 x 10 - 12**

Cycle 23

Push (A) Strength

Incline Dumbbell Press: **5 x 4 – 6**

Dumbbell Bench Press: **5 x 4 – 6**

Standing Barbell overhead shoulder press: **5 x 4 – 6**

Close grip bench press: **5 x 4 - 6**

Pull (A) Strength

Barbell Bent over row: **5 x 4 - 6**

Wide grip Weighted Pull-up: **5 x 4-6**

Barbell shrug: **5 x 4-6**

Dumbbell curl: **5 x 4-6**

Legs (A) Strength

Front Squat: **5 x 4 - 6**

Stiff leg deadlift: **5 x 4-6**

Seated calf raise: **5 x 4 – 6**

Standing barbell calf raise: **5 x 4-6**

Push (B) Size

Bench Press: **5 x 6 – 8**

Incline Bench Press: **5 x 8 – 10**

Cable Flyes: **5 x 12 – 15**

Seated dumbbell Shoulder Press: **5 x 8 – 10**

Smith machine Upright Row: **5 x 8 - 10**

Cable Lateral Raise: **5 x 12 - 15**

Weighted dip **5 x 8 - 10**

Tricep pushdown: **4 x 8 -10**

Pull (B) Size

T-Bar row: **5 x 6-8**

Wide grip Lat pull-down: **5 x 8-10**

Dumbbell row: **5 x 8– 10**

Barbell curls: **5 x 8- 10**

Incline dumbbell curl: **5 x 8 - 10**

Legs (B) Size

Hack Squat: **5 x 6-8**

Leg Press: **5 x 8 - 10**

Leg Curl: **5 x 8 -10**

Leg Extension: **5 x 8-10**

Standing barbell calf raise: **5 x 12-15**

Seated calf raise: **5 x 12 – 15**

Cable crunch: **5 x 10-12**

Hanging Leg Raises: **5 x 10 – 12**

Cycle 24

(Increase the weight on all exercises by 5-10%)

Push (A) Strength

Incline Dumbbell Press: **3 x 4 – 6**

Dumbbell Bench Press: **3 x 4 – 6**

Standing Barbell overhead shoulder press: **3 x 4 – 6**

Close grip bench press: **3 x 4 - 6**

Pull (A) Strength

Barbell Bent over row: **3 x 4 - 6**

Wide grip Weighted Pull-up: **3 x 4-6**

Barbell shrug: **3 x 4-6**

Dumbbell curl: **3 x 4-6**

Legs (A) Strength

Front Squat: **3 x 4 - 6**

Stiff leg deadlift: **3 x 4-6**

Seated calf raise: **3 x 4 – 6**

Standing barbell calf raise: **3 x 4-6**

Push (B) Size

Bench Press: **3 x 6 – 8**

Incline Bench Press: **3 x 8 – 10**

Cable Flyes: **3 x 12 – 15**

Seated dumbbell Shoulder Press: **3 x 8 – 10**

Smith machine Upright Row: **3 x 8 - 10**

Cable Lateral Raise: **3 x 12 - 15**

Weighted **3 x 8 - 10**

Tricep pushdown: **3 x 8 -10**

Pull (B) Size

T-Bar row: **3 x 6-8**

Wide grip Lat pull-down: **3 x 8-10**

Dumbbell row: **3 x 8– 10**

Barbell curls: **3 x 8- 10**

Incline dumbbell curl: **3 x 8 - 10**

Legs (B) Size

Hack Squat: **3 x 6-8**

Leg Press: **3 x 8 - 10**

Leg Curl: **3 x 8 -10**

Leg Extension: **3 x 8-10**

Standing barbell calf raise: **3 x 12-15**

Seated calf raise: **3 x 12 – 15**

Cable crunch: **3 x 10-12**

Hanging Leg Raises: **3 x 10 – 12**

Cycle 25 (Deload)

Push (A) Strength

Incline Dumbbell Press: **1 x 4 – 6**

Dumbbell Bench Press: **1 x 4 – 6**

Standing Barbell overhead shoulder press: **1 x 4 – 6**

Close grip bench press: **1 x 4 - 6**

Pull (A) Strength

Barbell Bent over row: **1 x 4 - 6**

Wide grip Weighted Pull-up: **1 x 4-6**

Barbell shrug: **1 x 4-6**

Dumbbell curl: **1 x 4-6**

Legs (A) Strength

Front Squat: **1 x 4 - 6**

Stiff leg deadlift: **1 x 4-6**

Seated calf raise: **1 x 4 – 6**

Standing barbell calf raise: **1 x 4-6**

Push (B) Size

Bench Press: **1 x 6 – 8**

Incline Bench Press: **1 x 8 – 10**

Cable Flyes: **1 x 12 – 15**

Seated dumbbell Shoulder Press: **1 x 8 – 10**

Smith machine Upright Row: **1 x 8 - 10**

Cable Lateral Raise: **1 x 12 - 15**

Weighted dip **1 x 8 - 10**

Tricep pushdown: **1 x 8 -10**

Pull (B) Size

T-Bar row: **1 x 6-8**

Wide grip Lat pull-down: **1 x 8-10**

Dumbbell row: **1 x 8– 10**

Barbell curls: **1 x 8- 10**

Incline dumbbell curl: **1 x 8 - 10**

Legs (B) Size

Hack Squat: **1 x 6-8**

Leg Press: **1 x 8 - 10**

Leg Curl: **1 x 8 -10**

Leg Extension: **1 x 8-10**

Standing barbell calf raise: **1 x 12-15**

Seated calf raise: **1 x 12 – 15**

Cable crunch: **1 x 10-12**

Hanging Leg Raises: **1 x 10 - 12**

Congratulations, you have finished the program. Take your measurements and photos again and compare them to when you first started, you should see a huge change!

Where to go from here?

Well that's up to you!

With this program you've seen what it takes to build a substantial amount of muscle. You could decide to start the program again and turn it into a 52 week long program or you can try something new. Hopefully you'll carry over the principals you've learned along the way to ensure you're always successful, no matter what workout program you follow. Whatever the case I created this book to empower you to reach your goals and I hope it has done just that.

Thanks again for purchasing this book and I hope to hear about your amazing transformation!

Best Wishes

Jason Farley.

Printed in Great Britain
by Amazon